Autoimmune Cookbook

Autoimmune All-Day Recipes Vol. 3

All Rights Reserved. No part of this publication may be reproduced in any form or by any means, including scanning, photocopying, or otherwise without prior written permission of the copyright holder. Copyright © 2014

About the Author – Melissa Groves

Melissa graduated from Hofstra University with a BA in English and Dance. As a dancer, she was always interested in nutrition and how to make healthy foods taste good. For over 15 years, he had a successful career in NYC as an advertising copywriter, but decided to leave that world to pursue her true passion, nutrition. She currently lives in New Hampshire, where she is going back to school, with the goal of becoming a registered dietitian. She is a 2000 graduate of the Institute for Integrative Nutrition. Her recipes have won national awards.

Table of Contents

Why the Autoimmune Protocol?

Foods to Avoid

Introduction

Chapter 1 – **Breakfast**

Blueberry-Banana Parfait

Strawberry-Kiwi Parfait

Tropical Fruit Cocktail

Quick Pumpkin Porridge

Sausage Hash

Chapter 2 – **Lunch**

Chilled Borscht

Creamy Cauliflower Soup

Potato-free Leek Soup

Vietnamese Chicken Wraps

Vegetarian "Sushi"

Crab-Stuffed Avocados

Caesar Salad

Cilantro Salmon Salad

Pineapple Tuna Salad

Shrimp with Raspberry Vinaigrette

Chapter 3 – **Dinner**

Shrimp Stir-Fry

Seared Scallops with Spinach

Swordfish with Pesto

Turkey Lasagna

Sweet Potato Shepherd's Pie

Beef & Mushroom Casserole

Beef Stir-Fry

Sausage & Sauerkraut

Lamb Roast

Liver & Onions

Chapter 4 – **Snacks**

Sardine & Avocado on Endives

Smoked Salmon Bites

Carrot Dip with Crudités

Rainbow Trifle with Whipped Cream

Key Lime Mousse

Why the Autoimmune Protocol?

Every day, dozens of people across the country get diagnosed with one or more autoimmune condition: systemic lupus erythematosus, celiac disease, Graves' disease, rheumatoid arthritis, type 1 diabetes... All these conditions and many more are caused by a dysfunction of the immune system. Normally, the immune system is responsible for fighting off microorganisms such as viruses, bacteria and fungi that would otherwise invade our bodies. However, some people's immune system has difficulty differentiating between self and non-self. Essentially, these people's immune system attacks their own body tissues. Some auto-immune diseases destroy the intestines, while others destroy joints, organs, skin or glands.

Science doesn't know the exact reasons why some people's immune system will attack healthy body tissues. What we do know is that many autoimmune reactions are in fact a response to a trigger: drugs, viruses or bacteria, irritants, food, etc. For example, someone with celiac disease will suffer intestinal damage after eating food that contains gluten (a protein found in wheat, barley and rye). Other people are sensitive to specific vegetables, chemicals or environmental triggers that cause heavy inflammation in their joints. In other words, autoimmune conditions seem to be similar to allergies, but with chronic consequences rather than an immediate reactions such as those seen when people come in contact with allergens. This leads the scientific community to further try to understand the role of inflammation in autoimmunity.

There are strong beliefs that some specific foods are more likely to trigger autoimmune reactions. These foods contain certain toxins, proteins or molecules that cause inflammation and trigger autoimmune reactions. This interesting topic has led to the creation of a very restrictive diet designed to eliminate all the common inflammation-causing "problem foods" from one's diet and reintroduce them one at a time in order to identify the culprit(s). This diet is known as the autoimmune protocol (AIP). The goal of the autoimmune protocol is to allow the person's immune system to rest, lower inflammation levels and allow for recovery. Once inflammation levels are low enough and the gut is healed, the person can start reintroducing foods one by one, carefully monitoring any resulting autoimmune flare-ups. Since the autoimmune protocol is generally pretty boring, most people are excited to reintroduce foods after several weeks.

It is important to *avoid cheating* while on the AIP. A small slip-up could ruin your efforts at trying to figure out which foods are causing your immune system to attack your own body. Healing from the damage done by inflammation is extremely important: chronic inflammation can lead to pain, loss of mobility, organ failure and several other potentially serious complications. Inflammation is the result of the immune system's attempt at eradicating a "threat" (the food you're eating) by launching a generalized inflammation attack all over your tissues and organs. Most people feel significantly better on the AIP and many decide to keep an anti-inflammatory diet for the rest of their lives. The Paleolithic diet is a very popular follow-up to the autoimmune protocol because of its major health benefits on inflammation levels.

How should you reintroduce foods? The key is to start small. Have a bite, then have a large portion of it later the same day. You need to eat enough of it to create a response. If you haven't responded after 4-5 days, chances are that you have no antibodies against that specific food. It can be considered safe and added to your regular diet. If you react to a food, it needs to be banned as it will nearly always trigger your immune system, much like an allergic person will always react to peanuts/shrimp/pollen/etc. Reactions can widely vary in nature, from "brain fog" and lethargy to insomnia, depression and disease flare-ups.

The autoimmune protocol is a very basic diet. It consists of fruits, vegetables and meat. However, not all vegetables are allowed: a specific family of vegetables known as nightshades causes autoimmune reactions in a large amount of people. The nightshade family includes eggplants, tomatoes, peppers (sweet and hot kinds – even chilies and jalapeños), mustard and potatoes. Artificial and no-calorie sweeteners are banned, as are processed foods, vegetable oils, dairy, grains, nuts, seeds, legumes, eggs, dried fruit and alcohol. What you can eat: meat (preferably grass-fed), fish and seafood, around 2 pieces of fruit per day, the occasional use of natural sweeteners (maple syrup, honey) in small amounts, fermented foods, many coconut products including milk, oil and coconut aminos, clarified butter (known as ghee) and non-nightshade veggies. Fats such as olive oil, lard and bacon fat are allowed, as are avocadoes, herbs, green tea and vinegar.

Since sticking to the autoimmune protocol is the key to its success, it is important to gather as much information as possible before starting. Of course, a cookbook containing creative autoimmune-friendly recipes is also a handy addition to your kitchen, as you will soon realize that you can't cook most of your favorite meals. Having such a cookbook can make following AIP guidelines easier as well. You can make AIP meals enjoyable by thinking outside the box and this cookbook is here to accomplish just that: inspire you to create healthy, anti-inflammatory meals that will make you feel truly great.

Foods to Avoid

You will want to avoid:

- Anything pre-packaged, canned or boxed, including frozen entrees and prepared salads or sandwiches. Most pre-packaged foods contain foods to avoid and are heavily processed. Canned or frozen veggies (excluding tomatoes) and pre-packaged baby spinach or lettuce mixes are generally fine
- No-calorie sweeteners and sugar substitutes, including stevia, xylitol and other sugar alcohols, sucralose, aspartame, acesulfame-k
- Added sugar (soda, candy and chocolate are obvious, but sugar is in everything including vinaigrettes and canned vegetables)
- All grains: wheat, barley, rye, rice, quinoa, amaranth, buckwheat, wild rice, oats, kamut, millet, sorghum, etc.
- Dairy, including butter, cheese, milk and yogurt. The *only* exception is cultured ghee (clarified butter, certified free of casein and lactose)
- Alcohol and excess caffeine (green tea is fine)
- Eggs
- Legumes: all dried beans, chickpeas, soy, edamame, hummus, etc. Green and string beans are fine
- Nuts and their oils
- Seeds and their oils: chia, flax, hemp, seed-based spices such as cumin and coriander, mustard, nutmeg, caraway, poppyseed

- Dried fruit and fructose (2 pieces of fresh fruit per day are acceptable)
- Nightshades: potatoes, tomatoes, sweet peppers (green, yellow, red, orange), hot peppers, chilies, eggplant
- Vegetable oils, except olive and coconut

Chapter 1

Breakfast

Blueberry-Banana Parfait

Prep Time: 5 minutes

Cook Time: N/A

Servings: 1

INGREDIENTS

1 large banana

1 cup blueberries

1 can full-fat coconut milk, refrigerated

2 Tablespoons shredded coconut, toasted

1 teaspoon ground cinnamon

INSTRUCTIONS

1. Take the coconut milk out of the refrigerator. Spoon the thick coconut "cream" out of the can to a small bowl.
2. Fold the cinnamon into the coconut cream.
3. In a bowl or parfait cup, layer 1/3 of the coconut cream, then half of the blueberries and bananas.
4. Add another 1/3 of the cream, then the other half of the blueberries and bananas.
5. Fill the cup with the remaining cream. Top with toasted coconut.

Strawberry-Kiwi Parfait

Prep Time: 5 minutes

Cook Time: N/A

Servings: 1

INGREDIENTS

1 cup strawberries, sliced

3 kiwi fruits, peeled and diced

1 can full-fat coconut milk, refrigerated

1 lime, juiced (about 2 Tbsp)

2 Tablespoons shredded coconut, toasted

1 teaspoon ground ginger

INSTRUCTIONS

1. Take the coconut milk out of the refrigerator. Spoon the thick coconut "cream" out of the can to a small bowl.
2. Fold the ginger and lime juice into the coconut cream.
3. In a bowl or parfait cup, layer 1/3 of the coconut cream, then half of the strawberries and kiwi.
4. Add another 1/3 of the cream, then the other half of the strawberries and kiwi.
5. Fill the cup with the remaining cream. Top with toasted coconut.

Tropical Fruit Cocktail

Prep Time: 5 minutes

Cook Time: N/A

Servings: 1

INGREDIENTS

2 tangerines, peeled and diced

1 papaya, peeled and diced

½ pineapple, peeled, cored, and diced

1 banana, sliced

½ cup shredded coconut, toasted

INSTRUCTIONS

1. Combine all ingredients except coconut in a bowl.
2. Serve immediately, or chill overnight.
3. Serve in bowls topped with coconut.

Quick Pumpkin Porridge

Prep Time: 2 minutes

Cook Time: 10 minutes

Servings: 4

INGREDIENTS

2 15-ounce cans 100% pure pumpkin

1 can full-fat coconut milk

½ cup shredded coconut, toasted

1 teaspoon ground cinnamon

Pinch of sea salt

INSTRUCTIONS

1. Heat the pumpkin and coconut milk in a medium saucepan, until hot (about 10 minutes)
2. Add the cinnamon and salt, and stir thoroughly.
3. Serve in bowls topped with toasted coconut.

Sausage Hash

Prep Time: 10 minutes

Cook Time: 30 minutes

Servings: 4

INGREDIENTS

2 Tablespoons coconut oil

1 small yellow onion, diced

2 cloves garlic, chopped

16 ounces chicken sausage, chopped

1 large sweet potato, peeled and diced

2 cups baby spinach

¼ cup water

Sea salt to taste

INSTRUCTIONS

1. Sauté the onion in the oil in a large skillet over medium-high heat until light brown, about 5 minutes.
2. Add the garlic and sausage and sauté until meat is browned, about 10 minutes.
3. Add the sweet potato and water. Cover and cook until the sweet potato is tender, 10-15 minutes.
4. Add the spinach, and stir in until wilted.

Chapter 2

Lunch

Chilled Borscht

Prep Time: 15 minutes

Cook Time: 30 minutes

Servings: 4

INGREDIENTS

1 large yellow onion, chopped

3 garlic cloves, minced

1 celery stalk, chopped

4 medium beets, peeled and diced

4 cups chicken or vegetable stock

2 Tablespoons apple cider vinegar

2 Tablespoons olive oil

1 teaspoon sea salt

INSTRUCTIONS

1. Sauté onion, and celery in olive oil in a large stockpot over medium-high heat until translucent (about 4 minutes).
2. Add the beets, garlic, and salt to the pot. Cook, stirring for another 3-4 minutes.
3. Add the vinegar and broth. Bring to a boil.
4. Reduce heat to low, cover, and simmer for 25 minutes.
5. Puree the soup with a hand blender, or blender.
6. Chill for several hours, until cold.

Note: This soup can also be served hot.

Creamy Cauliflower Soup

Prep Time: 10 minutes
Cook Time: 20 minutes
Servings: 4

INGREDIENTS

1 large white onion, chopped
4 cloves garlic, minced
1 large head cauliflower, cored and chopped
4 cups chicken or vegetable stock
2 Tablespoons olive oil
4 strips bacon (optional)
1 teaspoon sea salt

INSTRUCTIONS

1. Sauté onion in olive oil in a large stockpot over medium-high heat until translucent (about 4 minutes).
2. Add the cauliflower, garlic, salt, and stock to the pot. Bring to a boil.
3. Reduce heat to low, cover, and simmer for 8-10 minutes.
4. While soup is simmering, pan fry the bacon strips (if using) until crispy.
5. Puree the soup with a hand blender, or blender.
6. Serve in bowls, crumbling the bacon on top.

Potato-free Leek Soup

Prep Time: 15 minutes

Cook Time: 40 minutes

Servings: 4

INGREDIENTS

1 large yellow onion, chopped

2 large leeks, cleaned and sliced

1 large rutabaga, peeled and chopped

1 large head cauliflower, cored and chopped

6 cups chicken broth

2 Tablespoons olive oil

4 strips bacon (optional)

1 teaspoon sea salt

INSTRUCTIONS

1. Sauté onion in olive oil in a large stockpot over medium-high heat until translucent (about 4 minutes).
2. Add the leeks to the pot and cook, stirring, until lightly browned.
3. Add the rutabaga, cauliflower, salt, and stock to the pot. Bring to a boil.
4. Reduce heat to low, cover, and simmer for 30 minutes, until rutabaga is cooked through.
5. Puree the soup with a hand blender, or blender.

Vietnamese Chicken Wraps

Prep Time: 10 minutes

Cook Time: 15 minutes

Servings: 2

INGREDIENTS

1 cup chicken stock

1 pound skinless chicken breasts

1 small head cabbage

1 large carrot, grated

½ cup mint leaves, chopped

½ cup cilantro leaves, chopped

1 cucumber, grated

1 clove garlic, chopped

2 Tbsp lime juice

2 Tbsp olive oil

INSTRUCTIONS

1. Remove 6 outer leaves from cabbage. Wash, pat dry, and put 3 on each plate. Shred the remaining cabbage.
2. In a shallow pan, poach the chicken in the stock until cooked through (about 15 minutes).
3. Allow the chicken to cool, then shred and mix with the cabbage, carrots, cucumbers, mint, cilantro, lime, garlic, and olive oil.
4. Divide the mixture between the cabbage leaves.
5. Roll up the cabbage leaves and serve.

Vegetarian "Sushi"

Prep Time: 20 minutes

Chill Time: 30 minutes

Servings: 2

INGREDIENTS

4 sheets of nori

2 avocadoes, mashed

1 large carrot

1 beet, peeled

1 apple

1 daikon radish

½ cup watercress

INSTRUCTIONS

1. Cut carrot, beet, apple, and daikon into long thin strips.
2. Place nori sheet flat on a hard surface, with the shiny side facing down.
3. Spread 1/4 of the mashed avocado evenly over the nori.
4. Place 1/4 of the vegetables in a long strip in the middle of the piece of nori.
5. Roll the nori tightly from one end to the other, using the avocado to help it "stick."
6. Repeat with the other 3 sheets.
7. Chill for about 30 minutes.
8. Cut the rolls into pieces with a sharp knife and serve.

Crab-Stuffed Avocados

Prep Time: 15 minutes

Chill Time: 30 minutes

Servings: 4

INGREDIENTS

½ pound fresh crab meat, cooked

1 small bunch chives, chopped

2 stalks celery, chopped fine

1 cucumber, peeled and diced

2 large ripe avocados

2 lemons, juiced

2 Tablespoons olive oil

1 teaspoon sea salt

INSTRUCTIONS

1. In a large bowl, mix the crab, chives, celery, and cucumber.
2. In a small bowl, whisk together the oil, half of the lemon juice, and salt. Combine with the crab mixture.
3. Halve and pit the avocados. Scoop out the avocado meat from the bottom center of each half to create a "bowl." Chop the avocado and add it to the crab.
4. Rub the remaining lemon juice on the cut surfaces of the avocados.
5. Fill each avocado half with the crab mixture.
6. Chill for about 30 minutes before serving.

Caesar Salad

Prep Time: 5 minutes

Cook Time: 12 minutes

Servings: 2

INGREDIENTS

2 Tablespoons olive oil

2 Tablespoons lemon juice

4 anchovies

4 slices of bacon, diced

1 clove garlic, minced

4 cups romaine lettuce, torn

1 cup radicchio, torn

INSTRUCTIONS

1. Heat 1 Tablespoon oil in a skillet and sauté bacon until cooked, about 4-5 minutes.
2. In a blender or food processor, combine the remaining oil, the anchovies, and the lemon juice.
3. In a large bowl, toss the lettuce with the dressing and bacon.

Cilantro Salmon Salad

Prep Time: 5 minutes
Cook Time: N/A
Servings: 1

INGREDIENTS

2 cups mixed greens
6-oz can salmon
3 scallions, chopped
2 celery stalks, chopped
½ cup fresh cilantro, chopped
2 Tablespoons lime juice
2 Tablespoons olive oil
Sea salt to taste

INSTRUCTIONS

1. In a small bowl, combine the salmon, scallions, celery, and cilantro.
2. In a small bowl, whisk the olive oil and lime juice.
3. Serve the salmon on top of the greens and drizzle with the lime dressing.

Pineapple Tuna Salad

Prep Time: 5 minutes

Cook Time: N/A

Servings: 1

INGREDIENTS

2 cups mixed greens

6-oz can tuna

3 scallions, chopped

2 celery stalks, chopped

1 cup fresh pineapple, diced

2 Tablespoons olive oil

2 Tablespoons lemon juice

INSTRUCTIONS

1. In a small bowl, combine the tuna, scallions, and celery.
2. In a small bowl, whisk the olive oil and lemon juice.
3. Serve the tuna on top of the greens and drizzle with the lime dressing.

Shrimp with Raspberry Vinaigrette

Prep Time: 10 minutes

Cook Time: 5 minutes

Servings: 2

INGREDIENTS

12 jumbo shrimp, cleaned, with tails off

4 cups mixed greens

1 large avocado, peeled and chopped

1 cup frozen raspberries, thawed

¼ cup olive oil

3 Tablespoons lime juice

½ teaspoon sea salt

INSTRUCTIONS

1. Sauté the shrimp in olive oil until opaque on both sides.
2. In a blender, process the raspberries, oil, lime juice and salt until liquefied.
3. Serve the shrimp and avocado on top of the greens.
4. Drizzle the dressing on top of each serving.

Chapter 3

Dinner

Shrimp Stir-Fry

Prep Time: 10 minutes

Cook Time: 15 minutes

Servings: 4

INGREDIENTS

1 large yellow onion, sliced

1 large head bok choy

2 large carrots, sliced

1 pound shrimp, cleaned, tail on

2 cloves garlic, chopped

2 Tablespoons coconut oil

1 lime, juiced

1 teaspoon sea salt

INSTRUCTIONS

1. In a large sauté pan, sauté the onion in the oil until translucent, about 4 minutes.
2. In the meantime, chop the bok choy stems into slices. Add them to the pan along with the carrot slices and shrimp. Cook for about 5 minutes.
3. Tear the bok choy leaves and add them to the pan. Cook for another 5 minutes until leaves are wilted and shrimp is pink.
4. Add the lime juice and salt, and stir quickly to combine before serving.

Seared Scallops with Spinach

Prep Time: 5 minutes

Cook Time: 15 minutes

Servings: 2

INGREDIENTS

1 pound large sea scallops

2 Tablespoons coconut oil

2 pounds baby spinach

4 cloves garlic, sliced

4 slices bacon, diced

Lemon wedges

INSTRUCTIONS

1. In a large, skillet, heat 1 Tablespoon of the oil until very hot. Add scallops and sear until browned on each side, about 3 minutes per side.
2. In a separate skillet, heat the bacon (if using) in the remaining oil. Add the garlic and spinach, and cook, stirring, until the spinach is wilted.
3. Place the spinach in the center of 2 plates. Arrange the scallops on top of the beds of spinach. Serve garnished with lemon wedges.

Swordfish with Pesto

Prep Time: 10 minutes

Cook Time: 10 minutes

Servings: 4

INGREDIENTS

2 pounds fresh swordfish steaks

2 cups fresh basil

¼ cup unsweetened shredded coconut

1 lemon, juiced (about 2 Tablespoons)

¼ cup olive oil, plus 1 Tablespoon

1 clove garlic

1 teaspoon sea salt

Lemon wedges for garnish

INSTRUCTIONS

1. In a large skillet, sear the fish in 1 Tbsp of the oil until browned on each side (about 5 minutes per side, depending on the thickness of the fish). Can also cook fish on a grill, if desired.
2. While fish is cooking, combine basil, coconut, lemon juice, olive oil, garlic, and salt in a food processor and process 30-45 seconds, until combined but still coarse.
3. Serve fish topped with pesto.

Serve with a green vegetable, such as roasted asparagus.

Turkey Lasagna

Prep Time: 20 minutes

Cook Time: 20 minutes

Servings: 4

INGREDIENTS

1 pound ground turkey

4 large zucchini, sliced thinly lengthwise

1 yellow onion, chopped

2 cups mushrooms, sliced

2 cups baby spinach

2 cups fresh basil

1 lemon, juiced (about 2 Tablespoons)

¼ cup olive oil, plus 2 Tablespoon

1 clove garlic

1 teaspoon sea salt

INSTRUCTIONS

1. Preheat the oven to 425 °F.
2. Sauté onions in 1 Tablespoon olive oil in a deep sauté pan or wok for about 3 minutes, or until translucent.
3. Add the mushrooms and turkey and cook, stirring frequently, until lightly browned.
4. While chicken is cooking, combine spinach, basil, coconut, lemon juice, ¼ cup olive oil, garlic, and salt in a food processor and process 30-45 seconds, until combined but still coarse.

5. Grease the bottom of an 8 x 10 inch baking pan with 1 Tablespoon of the oil.
6. Layer one-third of the zucchini slices on the bottom. Top with one-third of the turkey mixture, then one-third of the sauce.
7. Repeat the layers twice more, ending with the sauce on top.
8. Bake about 30 minutes.

Sweet Potato Shepherd's Pie

Prep Time: 10 minutes

Cook Time: 50 minutes

Servings: 4

INGREDIENTS

1 pound ground turkey

1 large onion, chopped

2 medium zucchini, chopped

2 large sweet potatoes, peeled and diced

1 teaspoon dried thyme

1 teaspoon dried basil

2 Tablespoons olive oil

1 teaspoon sea salt

INSTRUCTIONS

1. Brown the meat with the onion in a large skillet. Cook until meat is fully cooked, about 15-20 minutes.
2. In another stockpot, steam sweet potatoes for about 20 minutes.
3. Add the zucchini and spices to the meat and cook for another 5 minutes.
4. Preheat oven to 400 °F.
5. Drain the sweet potatoes and return them to the pot. Mash with a potato masher and mix in the olive oil and sea salt.
6. Transfer the meat to a large casserole pan and pat it down with a spatula.

7. Spoon the mashed sweet potatoes on top of the meat, and spread it evenly across the pan.
8. Bake for 30 minutes.

Beef & Mushroom Casserole

Prep Time: 15 minutes

Cook Time: 1 hour and 20 minutes

Servings: 4

INGREDIENTS

2 pounds ground beef

1 pound mushrooms, washed and halved

1 onion, chopped

1 large head cauliflower, chopped

1/2 cup beef stock

2 Tablespoons olive oil

1 teaspoon dried parsley

1 teaspoon dried marjoram

1 teaspoon dried rosemary

1 teaspoon sea salt

INSTRUCTIONS

1. Brown the meat with the onion, celery, carrots, mushrooms, and garlic in a large stockpot. Cook until meat is fully cooked, about 15-20 minutes. Add the beef stock, rosemary, and thyme and stir.
2. In another stockpot, steam cauliflower for about 20 minutes.
3. Preheat oven to 400 °F.
4. Drain the cauliflower and return it to the pot. Mash it with a potato masher. Mix in the olive oil and sea salt.
5. Transfer the beef mixture to a large casserole pan and pat down with a spatula.

6. Spread the mashed cauliflower over the top of the meat.
7. Sprinkle the parsley on top of the casserole and put it in the oven.
8. Bake for 40 minutes, until cauliflower starts to brown.

Beef Stir-Fry

Prep Time: 15 minutes

Cook Time: 15 minutes

Servings: 4

INGREDIENTS

1 pound raw beef strips

1 yellow onion, sliced

1 medium carrot, sliced

8 oz mushrooms, sliced

1 Tablespoon ginger, minced

2 cloves garlic, minced

2 bunches broccolini, chopped

2 Tablespoons coconut oil

1 lemon, juiced

INSTRUCTIONS

1. Stir-fry the beef in the oil in a large skillet or wok with the garlic and ginger for 3-5 minutes, until cooked.
2. Add the vegetables and cook, stirring frequently, for 2-3 minutes
3. Add the lemon juice to the pan and cook for 3 more minutes.

Sausage & Sauerkraut

Prep Time: 10 minutes

Cook Time: 45 minutes

Servings: 2

INGREDIENTS

4 pork Kielbasa sausages

2 Tablespoons olive oil

1 onion, sliced

1 green apple, grated

2 cups sauerkraut

INSTRUCTIONS

1. In a large skillet, sauté the onion over medium high heat until translucent (about 5 minutes)
2. Add the sauerkraut and apple, cover, and cook on low for 20 minutes.
3. In the meantime, cook the sausages in a separate skillet until fully browned (about 15 minutes), or grill, if you prefer.
4. Serve the sausages on top of the sauerkraut.

Lamb Roast

Prep Time: 20 minutes

Cook Time: 30 minutes

Servings: 4

INGREDIENTS

2 pounds lamb cutlets, rack, trimmed

2 large parsnips, peeled and sliced

2 large carrots, sliced

1 large onion, cut into 8 pieces (halve, then cut each half into fourths)

2 sweet potatoes, peeled and chopped

4 sprigs of fresh rosemary

2 Tablespoons olive oil

1 teaspoon sea salt

INSTRUCTIONS

1. Preheat oven to 400 °F.
2. In a large bowl, combine vegetables with oil and salt and toss.
3. Add the vegetables to a large casserole dish. Add the lamb. Place the rosemary sprigs on top of the lamb. Bake for 25-30 minutes.

Liver & Onions

Prep Time: 15 minutes

Cook Time: 25 minutes

Servings: 4

INGREDIENTS

2 pounds beef liver, sliced

1 large yellow onion, sliced

3 cloves of garlic, chopped

8 oz sliced mushrooms

6 slices of bacon

1 teaspoon sea salt

1 teaspoon dried rosemary

1 teaspoon dried parsley

1 teaspoon thyme

INSTRUCTIONS

1. In a large skillet, brown the bacon.
2. Add the garlic and onions to the skillet. Cook until onions are translucent.
3. Add the mushrooms and spices and cook, stirring, for about 5 minutes. Remove the bacon mixture to a bowl.
4. In the same skillet, sear the liver for 1-2 minutes on each side.
5. Add the mushroom and bacon mixture back to the pan, cover, and cook over medium low for 5-10 minutes.

Chapter 4

Snacks

Sardine & Avocado on Endives

Prep Time: 5 minutes
Cook Time:
Servings: 4

INGREDIENTS

1-2 bunches endives
1 tin sardines in olive oil
1 Tablespoon apple cider vinegar
1 Tablespoon lemon juice
2 Tablespoons fresh parsley
1 avocado, halved, pitted, and chopped
½ teaspoon sea salt

INSTRUCTIONS

1. In a medium bowl, combine the sardines, vinegar, parsley, and lemon juice. Marinate the sardines for about 30 minutes in the refrigerator.
2. In the meantime, remove the leaves from the endives, wash them, and pat them dry. Set them on a platter, with the "cup" side facing up.
3. After the sardines are chilled, mix in the avocados. Use a spoon to divide the mixture among the endive leaves. There should be enough mixture to fill about 12 leaves.

Smoked Salmon Bites

Prep Time: 10 minutes

Cook Time: N/A

Servings: 2

INGREDIENTS

1 large seedless cucumber

4 oz smoked salmon

1 avocado

½ red onion

1 Tablespoon lemon juice

1/2 teaspoon sea salt

Chives for garnish (optional)

INSTRUCTIONS

1. Slice the cucumber into ¾-inch thick slices.
2. Slice the smoked salmon into 1-inch by 1-inch pieces.
3. In a small bowl, mash the avocado with the salt, lemon juice, and onion.
4. Spread the avocado mash evenly across each of the cucumber slices.
5. Top each cucumber with a piece of the smoked salmon.
6. Garnish with a chive, if desired.

Carrot Dip with Crudités

Prep Time: 10 minutes

Cook Time: 10 minutes

Servings: 4

INGREDIENTS

1 pound carrots, cut into 1-inch chunks

2 Tablespoons coconut oil

1 clove garlic, minced

1 teaspoon ginger, minced

½ teaspoon sea salt

1 Tablespoon lemon juice

Crudités for serving: Broccoli or Cauliflower florets, Sliced Jicama, Asparagus, Green beans, Cucumber spears, etc.

INSTRUCTIONS

1. Bring a small pot of water to a boil and boil the carrots 8-10 minutes, until soft. Drain and rinse.
2. Add all of the dip ingredients to a blender or food processor and pulse to combine.
3. Serve the dip with a variety of crudités for dipping.

Rainbow Trifle with Whipped Cream

Prep Time: 10 minutes

Cook Time: N/A

Servings: 6-8

INGREDIENTS

1 cup RED fruit, sliced (sliced strawberries, raspberries, watermelon)

1 cup ORANGE fruit (nectarines, cantaloupe)

1 cup YELLOW fruit (pineapple, mango)

1 cup GREEN fruit (kiwi, green grapes, honeydew)

1 cup BLUE fruit (blueberries)

1 cup PURPLE fruit (purple grapes, blackberries)

1 can full-fat coconut milk, refrigerated

1 teaspoon ground ginger

1 teaspoon ground cinnamon

1 date, unsweetened

INSTRUCTIONS

1. Take the coconut milk out of the refrigerator. Spoon the thick coconut "cream" out of the can into a blender jar.
2. Add the banana, ginger, cinnamon, and date to the blender jar. Process until combined.
3. In a large glass bowl, mix the fruits.
4. Serve the fruits with the coconut-banana cream spooned on top.

Key Lime Mousse

Prep Time: 10 minutes

Chill Time: 1 hour

Servings: 4

INGREDIENTS

2 cans full-fat coconut milk, refrigerated

2 limes, juiced (about 4 Tbsp)

1 teaspoon ground ginger

¼ cup unsweetened coconut, toasted

1 date, unsweetened (optional)

INSTRUCTIONS

1. Take the coconut milk out of the refrigerator. Flip cans over and open from the bottom. Pour off the liquid into a separate bowl.
2. Add the thick coconut "cream" from the cans to a blender or food processor.
3. Add the lime juice and ginger, and date (if using), and blend until thick and creamy.
4. Spoon into 4 individual serving bowls and chill for at least 1 hour.
5. Serve topped with the toasted coconut.

www.ingramcontent.com/pod-product-compliance
Lightning Source LLC
Chambersburg PA
CBHW071728170526
45165CB00005B/2206